1

Table of Contents

Melanoma, which means "black tumor," is the most dangerous type of skin cancer. It grows quickly and has the ability to spread to any organ.

Melanoma comes from skin cells called melanocytes. These cells produce melanin, the dark pigment that gives skin its color. Most melanomas are black or brown in color, but some are pink, red, purple or skin-colored.

About 30% of melanomas begin in existing moles, but the rest start in normal skin. This makes it especially important to pay attention to changes in your skin because the majority of melanomas don't start as moles. However, how many moles you have may help predict your skin's risk for developing melanoma. It's important to know if you're in a high-risk group for developing melanoma skin cancer. Because of the fast growth rate of melanomas, a treatment delay sometimes may mean the difference between life and death. Knowing your risk can help you be extra vigilant in watching changes in your skin and seeking skin examinations since melanomas have a 99% cure rate if caught in the earliest stages. Early detection is important because treatment success is directly related to the depth of the cancerous growth.

BREAKFAST

1. Loaded Tofu Scramble

Prep Time: 15 Minutes

Cook Time: 20 Minutes

Servings: 4

Ingredients

- 2 tablespoons canola oil, or high heat oil of choice
- 1 small (8 ounce/227 gram) russet potato, diced into about ½ inch pieces
- 1 medium onion, diced
- 1 bell pepper (any color), roughly chopped
- 3 garlic cloves, minced
- 1 (14 ounce/400 gram) package extra firm tofu, drained and patted dry
- 2 cups roughly chopped kale leaves
- 2 tablespoons soy sauce1
- 2 tablespoons nutritional yeast flakes
- 2 teaspoons ground cumin

- 1 teaspoon ground turmeric
- 1 tablespoon hot sauce (such as Cholula) or to taste
- Black pepper, to taste
- Kala namak, to taste (optional - for eggy flavor)
- Toppings or accompaniments of choice

Instructions

1. Coat the bottom of a large nonstick skillet with the oil and place it over medium heat.
2. Give the oil a minute to heat up, and when it begins to shimmer add the potato.
3. Cook the potato, flipping occasionally, until the pieces are just fork tender and crisp on the outside, about 8 minutes2.
4. Add the onion to the skillet and cook it with the potato until it just begins to soften, about 3 minutes, continuing to flip everything occasionally.
5. Add the bell pepper. Cook everything for about another two minutes, until the pepper begins to soften up.
6. Push everything to the sides of the skillet and add the garlic to the middle. Cook the garlic for about 1 minute, until very fragrant.

7. Break tofu into bite-sized chunks and add it to skillet. Flip everything a few times with a spatula to mix the ingredients.

8. Cook the mixture for about 5 minutes, flipping occasionally and breaking up chunks of tofu as needed, until the tofu begins to dry up and crisp in spots.

9. Add the kale, in batches if needed, letting each batch wilt slightly before adding the next.

10. Stir in the soy sauce, nutritional yeast, cumin, and turmeric. Flip everything again to incorporate the ingredients. Cook for 1 to 2 minutes, until most of the soy sauce dries up and the kale has fully wilted.

11. Remove the skillet from heat and season the scramble with hot sauce, kala namak (or table salt), and black pepper to taste.

12. Serve with toppings and accompaniments of choice.

2. Matcha Pistachio Muffins

Prep Time: 10 Minutes

Cook Time: 20 Minutes

Servings: 9-12

Ingredients

- 2 cups all-purpose flour
- ½ cup organic granulated sugar, plus 2 teaspoons for topping
- 1 tablespoon ceremonial grade matcha
- 2 teaspoons baking powder
- ½ teaspoon baking soda
- 1 teaspoon ground cinnamon
- ¼ teaspoon ground nutmeg
- 1 teaspoon lemon zest
- ½ teaspoon salt
- 1 cup unflavored and unsweetened non-dairy milk (room temperature)
- ⅓ cup canola oil
- 2 teaspoons lemon juice
- 2 teaspoons vanilla extract
- ½ cup shelled roasted and salted pistachios, roughly chopped

Instructions

1. Preheat the oven to 400°F and line 9 to 12 cups of a muffin tin with papers.

2. Whisk the flour, ½ cup of sugar, matcha, baking powder, baking soda, cinnamon, nutmeg, lemon zest, and salt together in a large mixing bowl.

3. In a separate bowl or large liquid measuring cup, stir together the milk, oil, lemon juice, and vanilla.

4. Pour the milk mixture into the flour mixture and stir just until combined.

5. Divide the batter among the prepared muffin cups. Sprinkle the pistachios on top, followed by 2 teaspoons of sugar.

6. Bake the muffins for 15 to 19 minutes, until a toothpick inserted into the center of a muffin comes out clean.

7. Place the muffin tin on a cooling rack and allow the muffins to cool before removing them from the tin.

Prep Time: 2hrs 10 Minutes

Cook Time: 30 Minutes

Servings: 12

Ingredients

- 1 cup unsweetened and unflavored non-dairy milk, warmed to 100-110°F
- 2 teaspoons organic granulated sugar
- 1 (¼ ounce or 7 gram) packet active-dry yeast
- 3 ½ cups all-purpose flour, divided, plus more for dusting
- 1 teaspoon salt
- 3 tablespoons vegan butter, melted and cooled, plus more for oiling the bowl and skillet
- Cornmeal, for coating the muffins

Instructions

1. Whisk the milk, sugar and yeast together in a small container or liquid measuring cup. Let the mixture sit for 5 to 10 minutes, until frothy.

2. While the milk mixture sits, whisk 3 cups of flour (reserving the last ½ cup) and salt together in a large mixing bowl.

3. Stir in the milk mixture and vegan butter. Continue mixing the ingredients until a soft dough forms, adding up to ½ cup of additional flour if needed.

4. Turn the dough onto a lightly floured surface and knead it until smooth and elastic, 5 to 8 minutes.

5. Place the dough into a lightly oiled bowl and cover it with a damp tea towel. Let the dough rise until doubled in size, 1 to 2 hours.

6. Turn the dough onto a lightly floured work surface and use a rolling pin to roll it to about ½ inch thick.

7. Cover a small plate with a thin layer of cornmeal and line a baking sheet with parchment paper.

8. Use a 3 ½ inch biscuit cutter to cut the dough into rounds. Dip both sides of each round in the cornmeal to lightly coat them, then place them on the baking sheet.

9. Cover the rounds with a damp tea towel and let them rise again until puffy, about 30 minutes.

10. Lightly butter the bottom of a large nonstick skillet or griddle and place it over medium heat.

11. Give the pan a few minutes to heat up, then place a few dough rounds on the hot surface. Cook them for 5 to 7 minutes on each side, until lightly browned and puffy.

12. Transfer the cooked muffins to a cooling rack to cool and repeat the cooking process until all of the dough rounds are cooked.

13. Use a fork to split each muffin in half without separating the halves.

14. When ready to serve, pull the muffin halves apart and toast them. Serve.

Prep Time: 10 Minutes

Cook Time: 10 Minutes

Servings: 10

Ingredients

- 3 tablespoons soy sauce
- 1 tablespoon maple syrup
- 1 tablespoon apple cider vinegar
- 1 teaspoon liquid smoke
- 1 (8 ounce or 227 gram) package tempeh
- 2 tablespoons canola oil (or high heat oil of choice)

Instructions

1. Stir the soy sauce, maple syrup, vinegar, and liquid smoke together in a small bowl.
2. Slice the tempeh, width-wise, into thin (approximately ¼-inch) strips.
3. Place the tempeh strips into a shallow dish and pour the soy sauce mixture over them.

4. Let the tempeh marinate for about 30 minutes. Gently turn the strips or use a spoon to drizzle some of the marinade over them once or twice while they soak.

5. Coat the bottom of a medium nonstick skillet with the oil and place it over medium heat.

6. When the oil is hot, add the tempeh strips in an even layer. Only add as many strips as you can fit without crowding. Cook the rest in a second batch.

7. Cook the tempeh strips for about 5 minutes, gently flip them with a spatula, and cook them for about 5 minutes more, until browned and crispy on both sides. Turn or shift the pan a couple of times while the tempeh cooks to ensure even heating.

8. Transfer the cooked tempeh strips to a plate. Cook the rest (if there are any) in a second batch, adding a bit more oil to the pan if needed.

9. Serve the tempeh bacon immediately.

Prep Time: 15 Minutes

Cook Time: 40 Minutes

Servings: 8

Ingredients

- 8 ounces dried mafalada pasta
- 1 cup raw cashews, soaked in water 4 to 8 hours, drained and rinsed
- 2 ½ cups unsweetened non-dairy milk, divided
- ½ cup organic granulated sugar
- ¼ cup cornstarch
- 2 teaspoons lemon juice
- 2 teaspoons vanilla extract
- 1 teaspoon ground cinnamon
- 1 teaspoon salt
- ¼ cup vegan butter
- ½ cup raisins

Instructions

1. Preheat the oven to 375°F and lightly oil a 2-quart baking dish.

2. Bring a large pot of salted water to a boil. Add the pasta and cook it according to the package directions.

3. While the pasta boils, place your cashews into a blender or food processor bowl with 1 cup of milk. Blend until smooth.

4. Add the remaining milk, sugar, cornstarch, lemon juice, vanilla, cinnamon, and salt. Blend again until combined.

5. When the pasta has finished boiling, drain it into a colander, then transfer it to a large bowl or back to the pot you boiled it in.

6. Stir the butter into the hot pasta until it fully melts.

7. Stir the cashew mixture into the pasta, then stir in the raisins.

8. Transfer the mixture to the baking dish.

9. Cover the baking dish and place it in the oven. Bake for 20 minutes, then uncover and bake for about 20 minutes more, until the top layer of noodles starts to brown.

10. Remove the dish from the oven and place it on a cooling rack to cool. The casserole will continue to set as it cools.

11. Serve the kugel warm. Divide onto plates and enjoy.

Prep Time: 20 Minutes

Cook Time: 40 Minutes

Servings: 6

Ingredients

- 1 (14 ounce or 400 gram) package extra firm tofu, drained
- 2 tablespoons soy sauce or tamari
- 2 tablespoons nutritional yeast flakes
- 1 tablespoon cornstarch
- ½ teaspoon turmeric
- 2 tablespoons olive oil
- 1 small russet potato, cut into ½ inch cubes
- ½ cup chopped red onion
- 2 garlic cloves, minced
- 1 small bell pepper, any color, diced
- 2 teaspoons ground cumin
- 1 teaspoon paprika
- ½ teaspoon ancho chile powder
- 1 cup cherry tomatoes, halved
- Salt or kala namak, to taste

- Black pepper to taste
- ½ cup chopped fresh cilantro

Instructions

1. Place the tofu, soy sauce, nutritional yeast, cornstarch, and turmeric into the bowl of a food processor and blend until smooth, stopping to scrape down the sides of the bowl as needed.
2. Preheat the oven to 375°F.
3. Coat the bottom of a medium (10-inch) oven-safe skillet*, with oil and place it over medium heat. When the oil is hot, add the potato.
4. Cook the potato until it begins to crisp, about 10 minutes, flipping it occasionally.
5. Add the onion and cook it with the potato for about 3 minutes more, until it begins to soften.
6. Add the garlic, bell pepper, cumin, paprika, and ancho chile powder. Continue cooking and stirring everything for about 2 minutes, until the garlic is very fragrant.
7. Remove the skillet from heat and stir in the cherry tomatoes and cilantro. Season the mixture with salt or kala namak and pepper to taste.

8. Scoop the tofu mixture directly into the skillet and fold everything together.

9. Bake until the frittata is set in the middle and browned on top, 30-35 minutes.

10. Remove the frittata from the oven and allow it to sit for a few minutes before cutting.

11. Serve with toppings of choice.

Prep Time: 10 Minutes

Cook Time: 55 Minutes

Servings: 10

Ingredients

- 1 ¾ cups all-purpose flour (whole wheat pastry flour works too)
- 1 teaspoon cinnamon
- ¾ teaspoon salt
- ¾ teaspoon baking soda
- ½ teaspoon baking powder
- 1 medium ripe banana
- ½ cup organic granulated sugar
- ⅓ cup coconut oil, melted (or your favorite baking oil)
- ¼ cup unflavored soy or almond milk, at room temperature
- 1 teaspoon vanilla extract
- 1 cup coarsely grated zucchini (about 1 medium zucchini)
- ½ cup raisins
- ½ cup chopped walnuts

Instructions

1. Preheat the oven to 350°.

2. Lightly oil an 8 or 9 inch loaf pan.

3. Stir the flour, cinnamon, salt, baking soda, and baking powder together in a medium mixing bowl.

4. Place the banana into a separate medium bowl and mash it with a fork or potato masher.

5. Add the sugar, oil, milk and vanilla extract to the banana and stir until well mixed.

6. Add the flour mixture to the bowl with the banana mixture and stir just until blended.

7. Fold in the zucchini, raisins and walnuts.

8. Transfer the batter to the loaf pan and smooth out the top with a spoon or rubber scraper.

9. Bake for 50 to 60 minutes, or until a toothpick inserted into the center of a loaf comes out clean.

10. Transfer the pan to a cooling rack and allow to cool completely before removing the loaf from the pan and slicing.

Prep Time: 1 Minutes

Cook Time: 25 Minutes

Servings: 4

Ingredients

- 2 tablespoons olive oil
- 2 medium leeks, white and pale green parts only, chopped
- 3 garlic cloves, minced
- ½ cup dry white wine
- 1 teaspoon dried thyme
- 2 pounds yellow potatoes (such as Yukon gold), peeled and cut into 2-inch pieces
- 3 cups vegetable broth, plus more as needed
- 1 cup full-fat coconut milk (from a can)
- Salt and pepper, to taste
- Chopped fresh chives, for serving

Instructions

1. Coat the bottom of a large pot with 2 tablespoons of olive oil and place it over medium heat.

2. When the oil is hot, add the leeks and sweat them, stirring occasionally, until they begin to soften, about 5 minutes.

3. Stir in the garlic and cook it with the leeks for about 1 minute, until very fragrant.

4. Stir in the wine and thyme. Bring the wine to a simmer and allow it to cook for about 4 minutes, until reduced by about half.

5. Stir in the potatoes, broth, and coconut milk to the pot. Raise the heat and bring the mixture to a simmer. Lower the heat and allow it to cook, uncovered, until the potatoes are just fork tender, about 15 minutes.

6. Remove the pot from heat.

7. Blend the soup with an immersion blender or transfer it in batches to a food processor or blender. You can leave some chunks in the soup or blend it until completely smooth, but be sure to stop blending as soon as it's as smooth as you like (don't overblend or it will turn gummy).

8. Return the soup to the pot if you removed it for blending, thin with additional broth if you'd like, and reheat it if necessary.

9. Remove the pot from heat and season the soup with salt and pepper to taste.

10. Ladle the soup into bowls and top with chives. Serve.

Prep Time: 10 Minutes

Cook Time: 15 Minutes

Servings: 4

Ingredients

- 3 tablespoons canola oil (or high-heat oil of choice), divided
- 6 corn tortillas, torn into bite-sized pieces
- Salt, to taste
- 4 scallions, white and green parts separated and finely chopped
- 2 garlic cloves, minced
- 1 small jalapeño pepper, seeded and minced
- 1 (14 ounce or 400 gram) package extra firm tofu, patted dry and crumbled
- 1 tablespoon soy sauce
- 1 tablespoon lime juice
- 1 teaspoon ground cumin
- 2 tablespoons nutritional yeast flakes
- ¼ teaspoon ground turmeric
- ½ cup tomato salsa

- Black pepper, to taste

- 2 cups refried beans (canned or homemade), warmed

- Toppings, such as cilantro, avocado, or shredded vegan cheese

Instructions

1. Coat the bottom of a large skillet with 2 tablespoons of oil and place it over medium heat.

2. Give the oil a minute to heat up, then add the tortilla pieces in a relatively even layer. Sprinkle them with a pinch of salt.

3. Cook the tortilla pieces for about 5 minutes, flipping them once or twice, until browned and crispy in spots.

4. Remove the tortilla strips from the skillet and transfer them to a plate.

5. Add the remaining tablespoon of oil to the skillet.

6. Give the oil a minute to heat up, then add the white parts of your scallions, garlic, and jalapeño pepper. Cook everything for about 1 minute, stirring constantly, until the garlic becomes very fragrant.

7. Add the crumbled tofu to the skillet and raise the heat to medium-high. Cook the tofu for about 5 minutes, flipping it occasionally with a spatula, until it begins to dry up and crisp in spots.

8. Add the soy sauce, lime juice, cumin, nutritional yeast, and turmeric. Continue cooking and flipping the mixture for 3 or 4 minutes longer, until most of the liquid dries up.

9. Return the tortilla strips to the skillet and stir in the salsa. Continue cooking everything for about a minute, just to heat up the salsa.

10. Remove the skillet from heat and season the mixture with salt and pepper to taste. Adjust any other seasonings to your liking.

11. Divide the refried beans onto plates and top them with the tofu mixture. Sprinkle with scallions and any other toppings you like. Serve.

10. Vegan Banana Walnut French Toast Casserole

Prep Time: 20 Minutes

Cook Time: 30 Minutes

Servings: 6

Ingredients

- 2 medium overripe bananas, peeled
- ¾ cup unsweetened and unflavored non-dairy milk
- ½ cup full-fat coconut milk (from a can)
- 2 tablespoons cornstarch
- 1 tablespoon maple syrup
- 1 teaspoon cinnamon
- 1 teaspoon vanilla extract
- ¼ teaspoon salt
- 2 tablespoons vegan butter, melted
- 4 tablespoons organic brown sugar, divided
- 6 cups bite-sized bread pieces (torn from a loaf of sourdough or French bread, preferably a day old)
- ½ cup chopped walnuts

For Serving:

- Vegan butter

- Maple syrup

Instructions

1. If you're planning on baking the casserole right away, preheat the oven to 400°F. Otherwise, wait to preheat the oven until you're ready to bake.
2. Place the bananas, milk, coconut milk, cornstarch, maple syrup, cinnamon, vanilla, and salt into a blender or the bowl of a food processor fitted with an s-blade. Blend until smooth.
3. Pour the butter evenly into the bottom of a 2 quart or larger casserole dish. Sprinkle the butter with 2 tablespoons of brown sugar.
4. Place the bread pieces into the casserole dish, then pour the batter evenly over the bread pieces. Gently stir the bread pieces to distribute the batter.
5. Sprinkle the walnuts over the casserole, followed by the remaining 2 tablespoons of brown sugar.
6. If you're planning on baking the casserole later, cover it tightly with plastic wrap and refrigerate for up to 12 hours. Remove the casserole from the refrigerator and remove the plastic before baking.

7. Place the casserole into the oven, uncovered, and bake it for about 30 minutes, until the top is crispy with dark brown spots.

8. Let the casserole sit for about 10 minutes before scooping or slicing portions and dividing it onto plates.

9. Top with vegan butter and maple syrup. Serve.

11. Vegan Mac & Cheese Soup

Prep Time: 10 Minutes

Cook Time: 20 Minutes

Servings: 4

Ingredients

- 1 ½ cups dry elbow macaroni
- 2 tablespoons olive oil (or high-heat oil of choice), plus a dash for the pasta
- 1 medium onion, diced
- 3 garlic cloves, minced
- ¼ cup all-purpose flour
- 1 (14 ounce of 400 ml) can full-fat coconut milk
- 3 cups unflavored and unsweetened soy or almond milk, plus more as needed
- 3 vegetable bouillon cubes (enough to make 3 cups of broth), crushed
- ⅓ cup nutritional yeast flakes
- 2 tablespoons Cholula hot sauce (or a similar vinegar-based hot sauce)

- 1 ½ cups fresh broccoli florets

- Salt, to taste

- Fresh chives, for serving

Instructions

1. Bring a large pot of salted water to a boil.

2. Add the macaroni and cook it according to the package directions.

3. Drain the pasta into a colander and return it to the pot. Toss it with a dash of oil to prevent sticking.

4. Coat the bottom of a large pot with the remaining 2 tablespoons of oil and place it over medium heat.

5. When the oil is hot, add the onion. Cook the onion for about 5 minutes, stirring frequently, until soft and translucent.

6. Add the garlic and cook it for about 1 minute, until very fragrant.

7. Add the flour and stir to form a paste that coats the onion. Cook the mixture, stirring frequently, for about 2 minutes.

8. Begin adding the coconut milk, a bit at a time, whisking between each addition to eliminate any

lumps from the flour. Stir in the soy or almond milk, bouillon, nutritional yeast, and Cholula.

9. Raise the heat and bring the liquid to a boil. Lower the heat and let the mixture simmer for about 10 minutes, until it thickens up a bit. Feel free to thin the soup with additional non-dairy milk if it gets too thick for your liking.

10. Stir in the broccoli and continue simmering for about 4 minutes, until the broccoli is tender and bright green.

11. Remove the pot from heat and stir in the pasta. Season the soup with salt to taste.

12. Ladle into bowls and optionally top with chives. Serve.

Prep Time: 10 Minutes

Cook Time: 30 Minutes

Servings: 4

Ingredients

For the Jackfruit Pulled Pork:

- 1 tablespoon canola oil, or high heat oil of choice
- 1 small onion, sliced into strips
- 2 garlic cloves, minced
- 2 (20 ounce or 567 gram) cans young green jackfruit in brine, drained and rinsed
- 2 tablespoons soy sauce
- ½ teaspoon liquid smoke
- ½ teaspoon smoked paprika
- Pinch cayenne pepper, or to taste
- 1 ½ cups vegan barbecue sauce
- Salt and pepper, to taste

For Serving

- 6 sandwich rolls
- Vegan coleslaw, or toppings of choice

Instructions

1. Coat the bottom of a medium skillet with oil and place it over medium-high heat.
2. Give the oil a minute to heat up, and then add the onion.
3. Cook the onion for about 5 minutes, stirring occasionally, until it softens and begins to brown.
4. Add the garlic and cook it for about 1 minute, until it becomes very fragrant.
5. Add the jackfruit, soy sauce and liquid smoke.
6. Cook everything for about 5 minutes, until most of the liquid cooks off. While the jackfruit cooks, use a spoon to being breaking up the large chunks.
7. Sprinkle the jackfruit with the smoked paprika and cayenne pepper. Stir a few times and continue cooking the jackfruit with the spices for about 1 minute.
8. Stir in the barbecue sauce.
9. Bring the sauce to a simmer, lower the heat and allow it to cook for about 20 minutes, stirring occasionally. You can add a splash of water if the sauce becomes too thick while cooking.
10. While the jackfruit simmers,take a couple of forks and pull the pieces apart to create a stringy texture.

11. The jackfruit is finished cooking when it is tender and stringy, resembling pulled pork, and the sauce is thick.

12. Stuff the pulled jackfruit into buns and top with toppings of choice.

13. Serve.

Prep Time: 20 Minutes

Cook Time: 40 Minutes

Servings: 2

Ingredients

- ½ cup brown rice
- 1 cup water
- 3 tablespoons soy sauce
- 1 ½ tablespoons rice vinegar
- 1 tablespoon maple syrup
- 1 ½ teaspoons toasted sesame oil
- 1 teaspoon freshly grated ginger
- 1 ½ teaspoons canola oil, or high heat oil of choice
- 7 ounces extra-firm tofu, cut into 1-inch cubes
- ½ cup frozen shelled edamame, thawed
- 1 cup diced fresh mango (about 1 medium mango)
- 1 cup diced red bell pepper (about 1 pepper)
- 2 small radishes, thinly sliced
- ½ avocado, sliced
- 2 tablespoons roughly chopped roasted macadamia nuts

- 2 tablespoons chopped scallions
- 2 tablespoons chopped fresh cilantro

Instructions

1. Place the rice and water into a small saucepan and set it over medium heat.
2. Bring the water to a boil, lower the heat and cover the pan.
3. Allow the rice to cook until tender and the water is absorbed, about 40 minutes, or according to the package instructions.
4. While the rice cooks, stir the soy sauce, rice vinegar, maple syrup, sesame oil, and ginger together in a small bowl.
5. Coat the bottom of a medium skillet with the canola oil and place it over medium heat.
6. Give the oil a minute to heat up, and then add the tofu. Arrange it in an even layer.
7. Cook the tofu for about 10 minutes, flipping once or twice, until browned and crispy on multiple sides.
8. Pour about a third of the soy sauce mixture over the tofu.

9. Continue cooking the tofu for about 1 minute more, until most of the liquid has cooked off.

10. When the rice has finished cooking, remove it from the heat and let it sit with the lid on for about 5 minutes.

11. Uncover the rice and divide it into bowls. Arrange the tofu, edamame, mango, bell pepper, radishes, and avocado over the rice. Sprinkle with macadamia nuts, scallions and cilantro, then drizzle with the remaining soy sauce mixture.

12. Serve.

Prep Time: 15 Minutes

Cook Time: 40 Minutes

Servings: 4

Ingredients

For the Roasted Garlic Aioli:

- 2 medium garlic bulbs
- 1 tablespoon olive oil
- 2 ripe avocados
- 3 tablespoons lemon juice
- ¾ teaspoons salt, or to taste
- ½ cup fresh basil leaves
- 3-4 tablespoons unsweetened non-dairy milk, as needed

For the Roasted Veggies:

- 8 ounces cremini mushrooms, cleaned and sliced
- 1 medium broccoli crown, broken into florets
- 1 medium red bell pepper, sliced into strips
- 1 small onion, roughly chopped
- 2 tablespoons olive oil

- ½ teaspoon salt or to taste

- ½ teaspoon black pepper, or to taste

For the Sandwiches:

- 4 (6 inch) sandwich rolls, sliced open and optionally toasted

- Fresh basil

- Red pepper flakes, optional

Instructions

To Roast the Garlic (for the Aioli)

1. Preheat the oven to 425°F.
2. Use a sharp knife to cut the top off of each garlic bulb.
3. Place each garlic bulb on a sheet of foil, then drizzle it with about ½ tablespoon of olive oil.
4. Loosely close the foil to enclose the garlic.
5. Bake the garlic until the cloves are soft and lightly browned, about 30 minutes.

To Roast the Veggies

1. Line one large or 2 medium baking sheets with parchment paper.
2. Arrange the veggies on the baking sheet(s).

3. Drizzle the mushrooms with 1 tablespoon of olive oil, and split the remaining tablespoon of oil evenly among the rest of the veggies.

4. Gently rub the oil into the veggies to evenly coat them. Distribute them in even layers on the baking sheet(s), then sprinkle them with salt and pepper.

5. Place the baking sheet(s) into the oven with the garlic, and roast the veggies until tender and browned in spots, about 20 minutes.

To Make the Aioli

1. Remove the garlic from the oven when it has finished roasting, then open the foil and allow it to cool while you gather the rest of the ingredients for your aioli.

2. Place the avocado, lemon juice, and salt into the bowl of a food processor fitted with an s-blade.

3. Squeeze the garlic bulbs to extract the roasted garlic, then add the roasted garlic to the food processor bowl.

4. Blend everything until smooth.

5. Add the basil and thin with non-dairy milk to your desired thickness. Blend again until smooth.

6. Taste-test and add more lemon juice and/or salt if you like.

7. To Assemble the Sandwiches

8. Slather the insides of the rolls with aioli, then stuff with roasted veggies and sprinkle with basil and optionally red pepper flakes.

9. Serve.

Prep Time: 15 Minutes

Cook Time: 45 Minutes

Servings: 4

Ingredients

- 3 tablespoons olive oil, divided
- 8 ounces white button mushrooms, cleaned and sliced
- 1 medium onion, diced
- 2 medium carrots, diced
- 2 medium celery stalks, diced
- 3 garlic cloves, minced
- 5-6 cups vegetable broth
- 2 tablespoons lemon juice, plus more to taste (I generally use about 3 tablespoons)
- 1 tablespoon finely chopped fresh rosemary (or 1 teaspoon dried)
- 1 tablespoon fresh thyme leaves (or 1 teaspoon dried)
- 1 teaspoon lemon zest
- ½ cup dried orzo pasta
- Salt and pepper, to taste

Instructions

1. Coat the bottom of a large nonstick pot with 2 tablespoons of oil and place it over medium heat.
2. When the oil is hot, add the mushrooms in an even layer. Cook the mushrooms for about 5 minutes, gently flip, and cook for about 5 minutes more, until they're browned on both sides.
3. Remove the mushrooms from the pot and transfer them to a plate.
4. Add the remaining tablespoon of oil to the pot and give it a minute to heat up.
5. When the oil is hot, add the onion, carrots, and celery. Cook the veggies, stirring occasionally, for about 5 minutes, until they begin to soften up.
6. Add the garlic and cook for about 1 minute more, until very fragrant.
7. Stir in 5 cups of broth, lemon juice, zest, rosemary and thyme. Return the mushrooms to the pot.
8. Raise the heat to high and bring the liquid to a boil.
9. Lower the heat to a simmer and allow the soup to cook for about 20 minutes, until the veggies are soft. Add more broth if the liquid reduces too much.

10. Stir in the orzo and continue to simmer, stirring occasionally, until tender, about 8 minutes (refer to package instructions).

11. Remove the pot from heat and season with salt and pepper to taste. Add more lemon juice if you like.

12. Ladle into bowls and serve.

Prep Time: 15 Minutes

Cook Time: 25 Minutes

Servings: 3

Ingredients

- 3 tablespoons vegan butter, divided
- 8 ounces homemade seitan (chicken-style, about half of a batch, can substitute store-bought seitan)
- 1 small onion, finely diced
- 1 garlic clove, minced
- 2 tablespoons all-purpose flour
- 1 cup water
- ½ cup unflavored and unsweetened non-dairy milk
- 2 tablespoons nutritional yeast flakes
- 2 tablespoons soy sauce
- 1 teaspoon white wine vinegar
- 1 teaspoon dried thyme
- ½ teaspoon rubbed sage
- Salt and pepper to taste
- 6 small slices crusty sandwich bread (or 6 larger slices, for larger sandwiches), toasted

- Chopped fresh chives and/or parsley, for serving

Instructions

1. If using homemade seitan, slice it as thin as possible, preferably using a mandoline slicer. If using store-bought, slice it thin as best as you can using a mandoline or sharp knife (depending on the size and shape of your seitan pieces).
2. Place 1 tablespoon of vegan butter in a medium skillet and melt it over medium heat.
3. Give the butter a minute to heat up, and then add the seitan slices. Avoid overcrowding the skillet, and cook the slices in batches if needed.
4. Cook the seitan slices for about 5 minutes on each side, until lightly browned, and then remove them from the skillet and transfer them to a plate.
5. Melt the remaining 2 tablespoons of butter in the skillet.
6. Add the onion and cook for about 5 minutes, until soft and translucent.
7. Add the garlic and flour, and stir well to coat the onions with flour. Cook for about 1 minute more, until the garlic becomes very fragrant.

8. Whisk in the water, milk, nutritional yeast flakes, soy sauce, vinegar, thyme, and rubbed sage.

9. Raise the heat and bring the mixture to a simmer. Lower the heat and allow it to simmer, uncovered, for about 10 minutes, until it thickens up a bit.

10. Return the seitan slices to the skillet and stir them into the gravy. Cook for about 1 minute more, just to heat up the seitan and give it a chance to absorb some gravy.

11. Remove the skillet from heat and season the gravy with salt and pepper to taste.

12. Arrange the bread slices on plates in pairs, and top with the turkey and gravy. Sprinkle with parsley and/or chives, and serve.

Prep Time: 20 Minutes

Cook Time: 20 Minutes

Servings: 6

Ingredients

For the Dressing

- ¼ cup olive oil
- ¼ cup red wine vinegar
- 2 garlic cloves, minced
- 1 teaspoon dried oregano
- ½ teaspoon organic granulated sugar
- ¼ teaspoon salt

For the Salad:

- 1 ½ cups dried orzo pasta
- Dash olive oil
- ½ medium red onion, coarsely chopped (about ⅔ cup)
- 1 cup Kalamata olives
- 1 medium cucumber, chopped (about 2 cups)
- 1 ½ cups grape or cherry tomatoes, halved

- ¼ cup chopped fresh parsley
- Salt and pepper to taste
- 1 batch tofu feta cheese

Instructions

1. Whisk all of the dressing ingredients together in a small jar or bowl. Set it aside.
2. Bring a medium pot of salted water to a boil. Add the orzo and cook it according to the package directions.
3. Drain the pasta into a colander, return it to the pot, and toss with a dash of olive oil to prevent sticking. Allow it to cool.
4. While the pasta cools, place the red onion into a small bowl and cover it with cold water. Allow it to sit for 10 minutes, then drain the water. (This will remove some of the onion's bite.)
5. When the pasta is cool transfer it to a large bowl. Add the onion, olives, cucumber, tomato, parsley and tofu feta. Pour the dressing over the ingredients and toss to coat.
6. Season with salt and pepper to taste. Serve.

Prep Time: 15 Minutes

Cook Time: 15 Minutes

Servings: 12

Ingredients

- 1 (14 ounce) can black beans, drained and rinsed
- 2 teaspoons ground cumin
- 1 tablespoon lime juice
- 1 garlic clove
- ½ teaspoon salt, or to taste
- ¼ cup fresh cilantro
- 3 large flour tortillas
- 1 ½ cups baby spinach
- 1 red bell pepper, finely diced
- ½ cup sliced black olives
- ½ cup chopped scallions (about 2 scallions)

Instructions

1. Place the beans, cumin, lime juice, garlic and salt into the bowl of a food processor fitted with an s-blade.

Blend until smooth, stopping to scrape down the sides of the bowl as needed.

2. Add the cilantro and blend for a few more seconds, until the cilantro is finely chopped and incorporated into the mixture.

3. Spread one third of the black bean mixture over one of the tortillas.

4. Arrange one third of the spinach over the beans, then sprinkle with peppers, olives and scallions.

5. Roll the tortilla up as tightly as you can. Then slice into 1-inch pieces.

6. Repeat for the rest of the tortillas and fillings.

7. Serve.

Prep Time: 15 Minutes

Cook Time: 15 Minutes

Servings: 2

Ingredients

For the Vegan Omelet:

- ½ cup chickpea flour
- 2 tablespoons nutritional yeast flakes
- 1 tablespoon ground flaxseed
- ¼ teaspoon baking powder
- ¼ teaspoon ground turmeric
- ¼ teaspoon paprika
- ¼ teaspoon black pepper
- ¼ teaspoon kala namak, or to taste
- ¾ cup water
- 1 tablespoon soy sauce or tamari
- 1 tablespoon vegetable oil
- For the Veggie Filling
- 1 teaspoon vegetable oil
- ½ medium onion, sliced and separated into strips

- ½ medium red bell pepper, sliced into strips
- 1 cup broccoli florets
- Salt and pepper to taste
- 1 garlic clove, minced

For Serving (pick your favorites)

- Cashew cream cheese, or your favorite vegan cheese
- Chopped scallions
- Hot sauce or ketchup

Instructions

Make the Vegan Omelets

1. In a medium bowl, stir together the chickpea flour, nutritional yeast, flax seeds, baking powder, turmeric, paprika, kala namak and black pepper.
2. Add the water and soy sauce and whisk until blended.
3. Allow the mixture to sit for 10 minutes.
4. Coat a medium skillet with oil and place it over medium heat. Pour half of the batter into the skillet. Cook the omelet until bubbles appear in center, about 4 minutes. Carefully flip and cook it for another 2 minutes.

5. Transfer the omelet to plate. Recoat the skillet with oil if needed and repeat with the remaining batter.

Make the Veggie Filling

1. Recoat the skillet with oil and raise the heat to medium-high. Add all of the veggies and stir-fry to desired tenderness, about 4-6 minutes.
2. Remove the skillet from heat and season the veggies with salt and pepper to taste.
3. Assemble the Veggie Stuffed Omelets
4. Stuff each omelet with cashew cream cheese and veggies. Fold over and top with toppings of choice.
5. Serve.

Prep Time: 30 Minutes

Cook Time: 30 Minutes

Servings: 4

Ingredients

For the Baked Tofu:

- 1 (14 ounce) package extra firm tofu, drained and pressed
- ¼ cup soy sauce or tamari
- 2 tablespoons rice vinegar
- 2 tablespoons maple syrup
- 2 teaspoons fresh grated ginger
- 1 garlic clove, minced
- 2 teaspoons sriracha (or to taste)
- 1 teaspoon toasted sesame oil
- For the Roasted Veggies
- 4 cups veggies of choice (see note), cut into bite sized pieces
- 1 tablespoon canola oil (or another high-heat oil)
- Salt and pepper to taste

For the Noodles:

- 8 ounces dried soba noodles
- 3 tablespoons soy sauce or tamari
- 1 tablespoon rice vinegar
- 1 teaspoon toasted sesame oil
- 2 garlic cloves, minced

For Serving:

- Chopped scallions
- Toasted sesame seeds

Instructions

To Make the Baked Tofu

1. Cut the tofu into 1-inch cubes.
2. In a shallow bowl, stir the soy sauce, vinegar, maple syrup, ginger, garlic, sriracha and sesame oil together.
3. Add the tofu to the bowl and gently stir to coat. Allow to marinate for at least 30 minutes.
4. Preheat the oven to 400° and line a baking sheet with parchment paper.
5. Arrange the tofu cubes on the baking sheet and place it in the oven.

6. Bake the tofu for about 15 minutes, flip and then bake about 15 minutes more, until the pieces firm up and darken.

To Make the Roasted Veggies

1. Arrange the veggies on a baking sheet or in a roasting pan or oven-safe skillet, and drizzle with olive oil. Toss a few times to coat.
2. Place the veggies in to the oven and roast just until tender, 12-18 minutes (time will vary depending on the type(s) of veggies used.

To Make the Noodles

1. Bring a large pot of water to a boil and add the noodles. Cook the noodles according to the package directions.
2. While the noodles boil, stir the soy sauce, vinegar, sesame oil and garlic together in a small bowl.
3. When the noodles are finished cooking, drain them into a colander, then return them to the pot.
4. Pour the soy sauce mixture over the noodles and toss to coat.

To Serve

5. Divide the noodles among bowls and top with roasted veggies, baked tofu, scallions and sesame seeds. Serve.

21. Vegan Soba Noodle Salad with Peanut Dressing

Prep Time: 20 Minutes

Cook Time: 10 Minutes

Servings: 5

Ingredients

- 1 (9.5 ounce or 269 gram) package soba noodles
- ½ cup creamy natural peanut butter
- 5 tablespoons soy sauce, plus more to taste
- 4 tablespoons lime juice, plus more to taste
- 4 tablespoons maple syrup, plus more to taste
- 1 garlic clove, minced
- 1 teaspoon freshly grated ginger
- ¼ cup water, plus more as needed
- 1 medium red bell pepper, sliced into strips
- 2 cups shredded red cabbage
- 2 medium carrots, julienne cut
- 1 cup frozen shelled edamame, thawed
- 2 scallions, sliced
- ¼ cup chopped fresh basil

- ¼ cup chopped fresh cilantro
- Toasted sesame seeds

Instructions

6. Bring a large pot of water to a boil. Add the soba noodles and cook them according to the package directions.
7. Drain the noodles into a colander and rinse them with cold water until completely cool. Let them sit in the colander for a few minutes to allow any excess water to drain.
8. While the noodles cook, make the dressing. Whisk the peanut butter, soy sauce, lime juice, maple syrup, garlic and ginger together in a small bowl. Thin with water as needed until the dressing is creamy but pourable.
9. Place the noodles into a large mixing bowl with the pepper, cabbage, carrots, edamame, scallions, basil, and cilantro.
10. Pour the dressing into the bowl and toss the mixture to coat everything with dressing.
11. Taste-test the salad and add more soy sauce, lime juice and/or maple syrup to taste.

12. Divide onto plates and top each with sesame seeds.

13. Serve.

Prep Time: 15 Minutes

Cook Time: 45 Minutes

Servings: 4

Ingredients

- 1 tablespoon olive oil
- 1 medium onion, diced
- 1 medium red bell pepper, diced
- 4 garlic cloves, minced
- 1 tablespoon chili powder
- 1 tablespoon ground cumin
- 1 teaspoon ancho chile powder
- 1 teaspoon dried oregano
- Pinch cayenne pepper, or to taste
- 5 cups cauliflower florets (about 1 medium head of cauliflower)
- 1 (15 ounce or 400 gram) can black beans, drained and rinsed
- 2 (15 ounce or 400 gram) cans fire roasted tomatoes
- ¼ cup tomato paste
- 1 ½ cups vegetable broth

- Salt & pepper, to taste

Instructions

1. Coat the bottom of a large pot with the oil and place it over medium heat.
2. Once the oil is hot, add the onion and pepper. Sweat the veggies for about 5 minutes, stirring occasionally, until the pepper is soft and the onion begins to turn translucent.
3. Stir in the garlic, chili powder, cumin, ancho chile powder, and oregano. Sauté the mixture briefly until it becomes very fragrant, about 1 minute, stirring constantly.
4. Stir in the cauliflower, beans, tomatoes, tomato paste and broth.
5. Raise the heat and bring the liquid to a boil. Lower the heat and allow the chili to simmer for 30 to 40 minutes, until the sauce is very thick and the cauliflower is tender.
6. Remove the pot from heat and season the chili with salt and pepper to taste.
7. Ladle into bowls and serve.

Prep Time: 15 Minutes

Cook Time: 40 Minutes

Servings: 4

Ingredients

- 8 ounces dried rotini pasta
- 2 tablespoons olive oil
- 1 medium onion, diced
- 3 garlic cloves, minced
- 1 (14 ounce or 400 gram) package extra-firm tofu, drained
- 1 teaspoon dried oregano
- ½ teaspoon fennel seeds
- ½ teaspoon red pepper flakes (or to taste)
- 2 ¾ cups canned tomato sauce
- 1 (14 ounce or 400 gram) can diced tomatoes
- 1 tablespoon balsamic vinegar
- ½ cup green olives (halved if they're large)
- ½ cup chopped fresh basil
- Salt & pepper, to taste
- Vegan Parmesan cheese, for serving

1. Bring a large pot of salted water to a boil and add the pasta.
2. Cook the pasta according to the package directions, until al dente, then drain it into a colander.
3. While the pasta cooks, coat the bottom of a large skillet with the oil and place it over medium heat.
4. When the oil is hot, add the onion. Sweat the onion for about 5 minutes, stirring frequently, until it becomes soft and translucent.
5. Stir in the garlic and cook it with the onion until very fragrant, about 1 minute.
6. Crumble the tofu into the skillet and cook it with the onion and garlic, stirring frequently, until it dries up a bit, about 5 minutes.
7. Stir in the oregano, fennel, red pepper flakes, tomato sauce, diced tomatoes, and balsamic vinegar.
8. Bring the mixture to a simmer, lower the heat a bit, and let it cook for about 10 minutes, until the sauce thickens up a bit, stirring occasionally.
9. Stir in the pasta, olives and basil. Cook everything a minute more, just long enough to reheat the pasta.

10. Remove the skillet from heat and season with salt and pepper to taste.

11. Divide onto plates, top with vegan Parmesan cheese, and serve.

Prep Time: 15 Minutes

Cook Time: 50 Minutes

Servings: 8

Ingredients

- 1 medium cauliflower head
- 2 tablespoons olive oil, divided, plus more as needed
- ¼ cup fresh parsley leaves, finely chopped
- 1 tablespoon fresh thyme leaves, or to taste
- 2 garlic cloves, minced
- ½ teaspoon salt, plus more to taste
- ½ teaspoon black pepper
- 2 tablespoons lemon juice

Instructions

1. Preheat oven to 400°F.
2. Using a large knife, cut the stem from the bottom of the cauliflower head to get a nice flat surface so it can sit upright.

3. Place the cauliflower head, cut side down, onto a baking sheet, oven-safe skillet, or in Dutch oven (Note 1). Slather the top with 1 tablespoon of olive oil. Cover the cauliflower with foil if using a skillet or baking sheet, or with a lid if using a Dutch oven.

4. Place the the cauliflower on the center rack of the oven to roast.

5. While the cauliflower roasts stir together the remaining olive oil, parsley, thyme, garlic, salt, and pepper in a small bowl (Note 2).

6. Begin checking the cauliflower after 30 minutes. Test it by inserting a sharp knife into the center. When the knife meets just a slight resistance, take the cauliflower out of the oven and uncover it. This can take up to 60 minutes.

7. Spoon or brush the parsley mixture over the cauliflower, drizzling it with some extra olive oil if needed.

8. Return the cauliflower to the oven, uncovered, and roast it for 10 minutes more, until the cauliflower is tender and lightly browned on the outside.

9. Remove the roast from the oven and carefully transfer it to a plate. Drizzle with lemon juice, then sprinkle

with additional salt and pepper to taste. Slice into wedges and serve.

Prep Time: 15 Minutes

Cook Time: 45 Minutes

Servings: 6

Ingredients

- 12 ounces dried spaghetti
- 1 tablespoon olive oil
- 1 medium onion, diced
- 2 medium carrots, diced
- 2 medium celery stalks, diced
- 4 garlic cloves, minced
- ¾ cup dry white wine
- 1 (28 ounce or 800 gram) can diced tomatoes
- ¼ cup tomato paste
- ½ cup unflavored and unsweetened non-dairy milk
- 2 tablespoons soy sauce
- 1 teaspoon dried thyme
- ½ teaspoon dried oregano
- 1 teaspoon organic granulated sugar
- 1 ½ cups cooked or canned (and drained) brown lentils1

- Salt and pepper, to taste

Instructions

1. Bring a large pot of water to a boil. Add the pasta and cook it according to the package directions.
2. Drain the pasta into a colander, return it to the pot, and toss it with a dash of olive oil to prevent sticking.
3. While the pasta cooks, coat the bottom of a large pot with a tablespoon of olive oil and place it over medium heat.
4. Give the oil a minute to heat up, then add the onion, carrots and celery. Sweat the veggies for about 5 minutes, stirring occasionally, until they begin to soften up.
5. Add the garlic and cook it for about a minute, until very fragrant.
6. Add the wine, bring it to a simmer, and let it cook until reduced by about half, about 4 minutes.
7. Stir in the tomatoes, tomato paste, milk, soy sauce, thyme, oregano, and sugar.
8. Raise the heat and bring the sauce to a simmer. Lower the heat and let the sauce simmer for about 30

minutes, until the veggies are tender and the sauce is thick.

9. Stir in the lentils and cook the sauce for a minute more, until the lentils are heated.

10. Remove the pot from heat and season the sauce with salt and pepper to taste.

11. Ladle over pasta and serve.

Prep Time: 20 Minutes

Cook Time: 35 Minutes

Servings: 4

Ingredients

- 6 ounces dried jumbo pasta shells (about 20 shells)

For the Quick Tomato Sauce:

- 1 tablespoon olive oil
- ½ large onion, diced
- 3 garlic cloves, minced
- 1 (28 ounce or 794 gram) can crushed tomatoes
- ½ tablespoon organic granulated sugar
- 1 teaspoon dried oregano
- ½ teaspoon salt, plus more to taste
- ¼ teaspoon black pepper, plus more to taste
- ½ cup fresh basil leaves, torn and lightly packed

For the Vegan Ricotta Florentine:

- ½ cup roughly chopped onion (about ½ of a medium onion)

- 3 garlic cloves, minced
- 1 cup raw cashews soaked in water 4-8 hours, rinsed and drained
- ½ cup unflavored and unsweetened soy or almond milk
- 2 tablespoons lemon juice
- 1 (14 ounce or 400 gram) package extra firm tofu, drained and broken into 5-6 large chunks
- ½ teaspoon salt, plus more to taste
- ¼ teaspoon black pepper, plus more to taste
- 2 cups fresh spinach leaves, coarsely chopped and lightly packed

Instructions

1. Bring a large pot of salted water to a boil. Add the pasta shells and cook them according to the package directions.
2. Drain the pasta into a colander, then return it to the pot and toss it with a few dashes of olive oil. Set aside.
3. Make the Quick Tomato SauceCoat the bottom of a medium saucepan with oil and place it over medium heat. Once the oil is hot, add the onion. Sweat the onion until softened, about 5 minutes.

4. Add the garlic and sauté it with the onion 1 minute more, until very fragrant.

5. Stir in the crushed tomatoes, sugar, oregano, salt and pepper. Bring the mixture to a simmer and lower the heat.

6. Allow the sauce to simmer, uncovered, for 15 minutes, stirring occasionally.

7. Stir in the basil and remove the sauce from the heat. Taste test and season with additional salt and pepper if desired.

8. Make the Vegan Ricotta Florentine

9. Place the onion, garlic, cashews, milk and lemon juice into bowl of food processor. Blend until smooth, stopping to scrape down sides of bowl as needed.

10. Add the tofu, salt and pepper. Pulse the machine until a thick and slightly chunky, ricotta-like texture is achieved, again, stopping to scrape down the sides of bowl as needed.

11. If some space remains in food processor bowl, add the spinach and pulse until finely chopped and well blended. Otherwise, transfer mixture to a bowl and stir the spinach in by hand.

12. Taste-test and season the mixture with additional salt and pepper to taste.

13. Make the Stuffed Shells FlorentinePreheat the oven to 400°. Coat the bottom of a 9 inch by 9 inch baking dish or 10 inch round oven-safe skillet with about half of sauce.

14. Stuff the shells with the ricotta mixture and arrange them in a single layer in the baking dish or skillet. Top with the remaining sauce.

15. Cover and bake the shells for 20-25 minutes, until the sauce is bubbly.

16. Remove the shells from the oven and allow them to sit for 5 minutes before serving.

Prep Time: 15 Minutes

Cook Time: 20 Minutes

Servings: 3

Ingredients

- 1 pound shelf-stable potato gnocchi
- 1 small bunch (6-8 ounces) lacinato kale, torn into small pieces
- 2 tablespoons olive oil, plus a dash
- ½ cup finely chopped shallots (1-2 shallots)
- 3 garlic cloves, minced
- 2 tablespoons all-purpose flour
- ¼ cup dry white wine
- 1 tablespoon fresh thyme leaves
- 1 cup full-fat coconut milk (from a can)
- ½ teaspoon salt (or to taste)
- 1 tablespoon lemon juice
- 1 teaspoon lemon zest
- Black pepper, to taste
- Red pepper flakes, for serving
- Vegan Parmesan cheese, for serving

Instructions

1. Bring a large pot of salted water to a boil.

2. Add the gnocchi to the pot and cook it according to the package directions. When you've got about 30 seconds of cook time left, stir in the kale and continue cooking until the gnocchi float the kale is bright green.

3. Drain the gnocchi and kale into a colander, return them to the pot, and toss them with a dash of olive oil to prevent sticking. Set aside.

4. Coat the bottom of a large skillet with 2 tablespoons of olive oil and place it over medium heat.

5. When the oil is hot, add the shallots. Sweat the shallots for about 5 minutes, stirring frequently, until they become soft and translucent.

6. Add the garlic and cook it with the shallots for about 30 second more, until it becomes very fragrant.

7. Stir in the flour. Continue cooking and stirring the mixture for about 2 minutes, until the flour forms a smooth paste and coats the shallots.

8. Stir in the white wine and thyme, and bring the liquid to a simmer. Allow the mixture to simmer for about 4 minutes, until the liquid reduced by about half.

9. Stir in the salt, then add the coconut milk, a bit at a time in order to smoothly incorporate it with the flour.

10. Bring the mixture to a boil, lower the heat and allow it to simmer for about 5 minutes, stirring occasionally, until it becomes smooth and thick.

11. Stir in the lemon juice, zest, gnocchi and kale. Cook everything for about 30 second more, stirring to coat the gnocchi and kale with the sauce.

12. Remove the skillet from heat and season the gnocchi with black pepper and additional salt to taste.

13. Divide onto plates and serve with red pepper flakes and vegan Parmesan cheese.

Prep Time: 15 Minutes

Cook Time: 15 Minutes

Servings: 4

Ingredients

- 10 ounces dried penne pasta
- 1 ½ pounds fresh asparagus spears
- Salt, to taste
- 2 tablespoons olive oil
- 4 garlic cloves, minced
- ⅓ cup balsamic vinegar
- ¼ teaspoon red pepper flakes (or to taste)
- Black pepper, to taste
- Chopped fresh parsley or basil (optional)

Instructions

1. Bring a large pot of salted water to a boil. Add the pasta and cook it according to the package directions, until al dente. Drain the pasta into a colander, return it to the pot, and toss it with a dash of olive oil.

2. Break the woody ends from the asparagus spears, then cut them into 2-inch pieces.

3. Add ½ cup of water to a large skillet and place it over high heat. Bring the water to a boil.

4. Lower the heat to medium and add the asparagus. Cover the skillet and steam the asparagus for about 2 minutes, until they just begin to tenderize and turn bright green.

5. Transfer the asparagus to a plate, then pour the water out of the skillet.

6. Return the skillet to the burner and coat the bottom with the olive oil. Raise the heat to medium-hight.

7. Give the oil a minute to heat up, then return the asparagus to the skillet and sprinkle it with a pinch of salt. Cook the asparagus for about 3 minutes, flipping once or twice, until it begins to darken in spots.

8. Lower the heat to medium. Push the asparagus to the sides and add the garlic to the center of the skillet.

9. Cook the garlic, stirring constantly, for about 1 minute, until it becomes very fragrant.

10. Pour the balsamic vinegar into the skillet, along with the red pepper flakes. The vinegar should start simmering right away. Let it cook for about a minute, to reduce slightly.

11. Add the pasta to the skillet and toss it to coat it with the balsamic. Cook everything for about a minute, until the pasta is heated throughout.

12. Remove the skillet from heat and season the pasta with salt and pepper to taste. Optionally, sprinkle with parsley or basil.

13. Divide onto plates and serve.

Prep Time: 15 Minutes

Cook Time: 25 Minutes

Servings: 4

Ingredients

- 1 tablespoon olive oil
- 1 medium onion, diced
- 1 red bell pepper, diced
- 1 poblano pepper, diced
- 4 garlic cloves, minced
- 2 teaspoons smoked paprika
- 2 teaspoons ground cumin
- ¼ teaspoon cayenne pepper
- 2 cups vegetable broth
- 1 medium russet potato, scrubbed and cut into ½-inch pieces
- 2 (14 ounce or 400 gram) cans chickpeas, drained and rinsed
- 1 (14 ounce or 400 gram) can fire roasted tomatoes
- 2 tablespoons tomato paste
- Salt and pepper, to taste

- Fresh cilantro and/or scallions, for topping

Instructions

1. Coat the bottom of a large pot with the oil and place it over medium heat.
2. When the oil is hot, add the onion, bell pepper, and poblano pepper. Sweat the veggies for about 10 minutes, until they soften and the onion becomes translucent.
3. Add the garlic, smoked paprika, cumin, and cayenne pepper. Cook everything for about 1 minute more, until the garlic becomes very fragrant.
4. Stir in the broth, potatoes, and chickpeas.
5. Raise the heat and bring the liquid to a boil. Lower the heat and let it simmer until the potato is fork tender, about 12 minutes, stirring occasionally. You can add some hot water to the pot if the liquid level becomes too low.
6. Stir in the tomatoes and tomato paste. Continue cooking everything for about 5 minutes more, until the stew is thick.
7. Remove the pot from the heat and season it with salt and pepper to taste.

8. Ladle into bowls and top with scallions and cilantro.
   Serve.

Prep Time: 15 Minutes

Cook Time: 40 Minutes

Servings: 6

Ingredients

- 1 cup small dried pasta shells
- 2 tablespoons olive oil
- 2 medium fennel bulbs, diced
- 2 medium carrots, diced
- 4 garlic cloves, minced
- ¾ cup dry white wine
- 6 cups vegetable broth
- 1 (14 ounce or 400 gram) can cannellini beans, drained and rinsed
- Pinch red pepper flakes, or to taste
- 1 tablespoon lemon juice
- ½ cup chopped fresh basil
- Salt & black pepper, to taste

Instructions

1. Bring a medium pot of salted water to a boil. Add the pasta shells and cook them according to the package directions. Drain them into a colander when done.
2. While the pasta cooks, coat the bottom of a large pot with the oil and place it over medium heat.
3. When the oil is hot, add the fennel and carrots. Sweat the veggies, stirring frequently, until they begin to soften up after about 10 minutes.
4. Stir in the garlic and cook it with the veggies until very fragrant, about 1 minute.
5. Stir in the wine. Raise the heat and bring it to a simmer. Let it cook for about 4 minutes, until reduced by about half.
6. Stir in the broth, beans, and red pepper flakes.
7. Bring the broth to a boil, lower the heat and let the soup simmer for about 20 minutes, until the carrots and fennel are tender.
8. Remove the pot from heat and stir in the pasta, along with lemon juice, basil, salt and pepper to taste.
9. Ladle into bowls and serve.